CONTENTS

Introduction 5

Fibronyms 9

Top Ten Lists 19

Limericks and more 31

What you say / What you mean ... 41

Famous Last Words - FLAWS ... 45

Personalized Greeting Cards.... 47

What If 51

Painecdotes 61

Parodies: Fibromyalgia songs 69

MiscellPAINey 85

How Bad Is My Pain? 95

INTRODUCTION

I first met Barbara Dawkins in the Spring of 1996 at a fibromyalgia seminar in Nashville, Tennessee. Since we both have fibromyalgia, we were never really strangers when we first met, and I quickly came to appreciate her great sense of humor. She told me she thought my book, "Laugh at Your Muscles" was funny, even after repeated questioning and clarification from me! And she even sang her fibromyalgia songs to me.

I like Barbara's use of humor to help ease the daily pain of fibromyalgia as I have always believed that laughter truly is the best medicine. Plus, Barbara has all kinds of funny material including fibromyalgia parodies, definitions, stories and miscellpainey that ultimately became chapters in this book.

We agreed to combine our material and co-author a humor book, "Laugh at Your Muscles, Two." We figured if each of us could get a half of a laugh, our combined efforts might generate a whole laugh!

For me, it has been fun co-authoring this book with Barbara and I am thankful for this opportunity. I hope you enjoy this light look at fibromyalgia and if you have any stories, ideas or other things you'd like to share, send them to Anadem Publishing and we'll put them all together for a future book.

Remember, you are supposed to laugh when you read this book, that's an official doctor's prescription!

Mark J. Pellegrino, M.D.
August 1997

My fibromyalgia introduced me to many wonderful people I would otherwise have never met, greatly enriching my life. I even met a distant cousin raised just a few miles from my childhood home — someone I'd never met before. While she grew up knowing my sister and brother, she didn't even know I existed!

My fibromyalgia has taught me to better distinguish between true friends and the users. While I've always known the difference, I tolerated disingenuous
people because I enjoyed helping others and enjoyed the things I did. When fibromyalgia made me need their help, I didn't expect a lot. But I was surprised by open hostility. After severing any vestige of emotional affinity for those people, I'm much happier and, in spite of having fibromyalgia, am much healthier without them.

When my husband, Wayne, was a preschooler, he had polio. We have attended several polio-related conferences. I was not diagnosed with fibromyalgia until almost two years after he retired because of post-polio syndrome (PPS). My fibromyalgia has enlightened me about why, many years ago, someone at a polio meeting picked *me* instead of Wayne as the person who'd had polio. One lady asked me if I wore a full leg brace with my polio. When I (tactfully, I hope) explained that Wayne was the polio survivor, she looked stunned and exclaimed, "I never would have thought it was him! He looks so normal!"

Now I also know why I identified with more symptoms mentioned by speakers at polio conferences than Wayne did. Many people with PPS develop FMS as well. It may be because the pain from post-polio interferes with the person's ability to get enough restorative sleep. If that person has a genetic predisposition for fibromyalgia, then that interference could trigger the cascade of FMS symptoms.

My fibromyalgia has taught me how to help my health care providers help me better. My fibromyalgia health care team now includes my family doctor, a physical medicine and rehabilitation specialist, physical therapist, massotherapist, pharmacist, rehabilitation counselor, and chiropractor. I can describe numerous types of headache pain and generally know which treatment will help each type. I'm glad I know these things but I'd rather not have a reason to need to know them!

Barbara Dawkins
August 1997

FIBRONYMS

Ambidextrous

The ability to be equally clumsy with both hands.

Crampgrounds

Outdoors arena where atmospheric conditions trigger flare-ups.

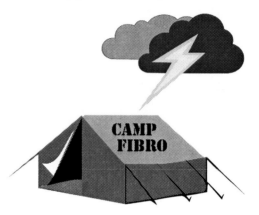

Dinosore

Extinct reptile that had FMS.

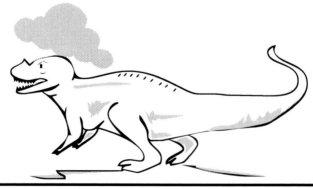

Endolphins

Sea mammals serving as natural pain killers when cavorting in your body.

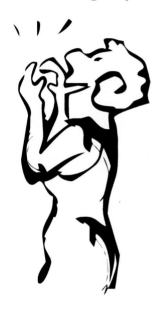

Etiquette

Knowing the proper way to tell people you've completely forgotten their name.

Expert

One who dosen't know any more than you do, but uses slides.

Fibrohug

A hug between two fibromites who wrap their arms around each other and use their fingers to massage each other's backs.

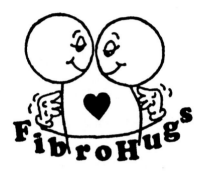

Fibromite

Person with fibromyalgia syndrome.

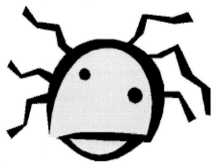

Hall of Pain

Museum immortalizing fibromites who have survived 50 or more years with fibromyalgia.

Hippocrampy

Section of brain felt to be responsible for causing fibromyalgia.

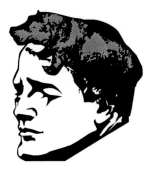

Leapfog

Fibro sport where fibromites make mental leaps over each other.

Miscellpainey

Collection of things related to various types of pain.

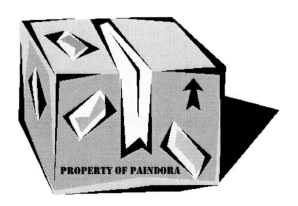

Opaingutan

Ape that has FMS.

Painapple

Tropical fruit that may trigger IBS or reactive hypoglycemia when packed in sugar.

Painclothesmen

Detectives who help fibromites find clothes that won't hurt them.

Painecdotes

Short narrative recounts of fibro pain.

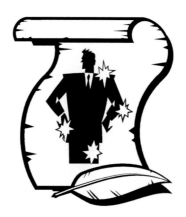

Painesthesiologist

Physician specializing in making patients lose the sensation of pain.

Painguins

Little known flightless birds thought to have FMS.

Painicillin

Antibiotic used in the treatment of FMS pain.

Painigree

A record of your ancestors who had FMS.

Painmanship

The way a fibromite writes.

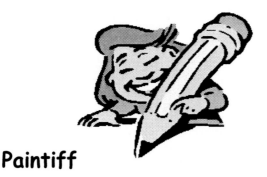

Paintiff

Legal term for persons who bring charges against someone who hit them and caused their fibromyalgia.

Paintomime

Fibromite who is in too much pain to speak so must use gestures to let the doctor know the locations of the symptoms.

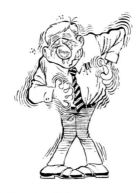

Porcupains

Sharp-spined animal that tap dances on fibromites in their sleep.

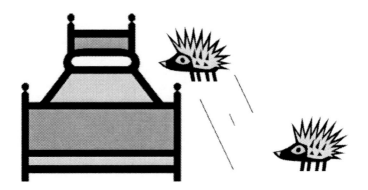

Postpainment

Delay between overdoing something and the pain from it.

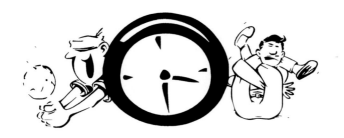

Refluxedo

Semiformal evening attire worn by fibromites with IBS.

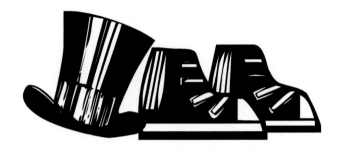

Retroflux

When the stomach makes an abrupt back flip.

Twitchcraft

Art of making all your muscles act up on cue.

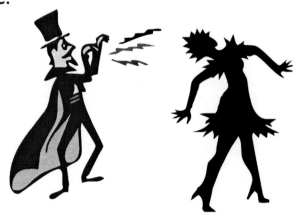

TOP TEN
LISTS

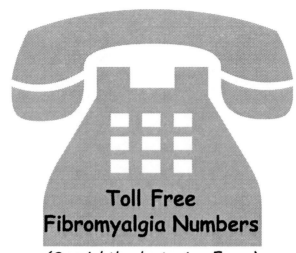

Toll Free
Fibromyalgia Numbers

(Special thanks to Ann Evans)

1. 1-800-IMI8418

2. 1-800-NEEDADR

3. 1-800-URAPAIN

4. 1-800-GOFIBRO

5. 1-800-IHURTIN

6. 1-800-TRIGGER

7. 1-800-VICODIN

8. 1-800-SURVIVE

9. 1-800-INAGONY

10. 1-800-MUSCLES

Signs That Your Child May Have Fibromyalgia

1. Has growing pains without actual growth.

2. Says your perfume makes him "puke his guts out."

3. Says when she grows up, will consider numerous jobs as long as they are classified as sedentary.

4. Only kid in school history to flunk gym.

5. Volunteers at school to be in a sleep study.

6. For Christmas, all he wants is a hot tub.

7. Selective memory loss (can't remember homework assignment).

8. Complains of constant hairballs in her throat.

9. Gets upset if you don't park exactly between the lines, gets completely embarrassed and refuses to get out of car if you straddle a line.

10. Spends more time in the bathroom than the classroom.

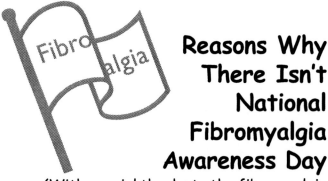

Reasons Why There Isn't National Fibromyalgia Awareness Day

(With special thanks to the fibromyalgia support group on the internet)

1. No one could remember the day.

2. "Things to do for the rally" list was too heavy for man or machine to carry.

3. FDA warnings about possible spontaneous combustion of too many people flared up at the same time.

4. No volunteers to carry the signs.

5. Concern the planned program wouldn't leave enough time to whine and complain.

6. Not enough bumper stickers: "See, I told you I was sick."

7. All the TENS units and magnets could short out the electrical systems.

8. Not enough port-a-potties for those with IBS.

9. Planning meeting never held because nobody's house was clean enough.

10. How could there be an awareness day for something that doesn't exist?

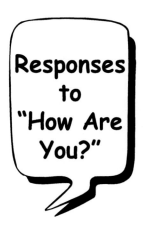

Responses to "How Are You?"

1. OUCH! Must you vibrate the air so much?

2. Like blender pulp.

3. Great! I think I found a spot that doesn't hurt!

4. Disillusioned. I thought I'd found a spot that didn't hurt.

5. Lower than the underbelly of a red bug.

6. Like a used fur ball.

7. Like 40 miles of bad road.

8. Like roadkill with buzzards circling.

9. Like a jellyfish in the Sahara.

10. Like a total eclipse of the brain.

Things to do With a Workout Video

1. Garbage can target practice

2. Tap your foot to the music

3. Enjoy the scenery

4. Critique the outfits

5. Search the house for it —
   Find it in the VCR

6. Sleep through it

7. Bury it

8. Plan a major melt down

9. Trade it in for a Happy Massager

10. Send it to "Mission Impossible"

Religious Songs

1. Been Through Enough

2. God Is Up To Something

3. God Will Make This Trial A Blessing

4. Hallelujah Anyhow

5. Help Me Stand, Lord

6. I'll Have A New Body

7. It Runs In The Family

8. Learning To Lean

9. Look What I'm Trading For A Mansion

10. Where Am I Going

Proven Cures for Fibromyalgia

1.

2.

3.

4.

5.

6.

7.

8.

9.

10.

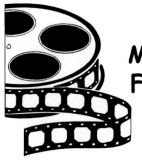

Movies about Fibromyalgia

1. Mutant Species

2. Clueless

3. Airheads

4. Sleepwalkers

5. Body Language

6. Necessary Roughness

7. Looking for Miracles

8. Silent Rage

9. The Fog

10. Hell Fighters

Things Fibromyalgia People Worry about
(Special thanks to Ann Evans)

1. Should I eat a microwave chicken dinner or microwave turkey dinner tonight?

2. What will I wear to my niece's 4th birthday party next week?

3. I need to reorganize my recycling bins soon.

4. Is the air pressure in my tires okay?

5. Will I be able to park the car exactly between the lines?

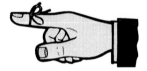

6. I think I forgot to floss a tooth this morning.

7. Have any foods in my refrigerator passed the expiration date today?

8. Why in the heck is my check book off 12 cents?

9. I better not be late for my doctor's appointment.

10. Should I change the message on my answering machine now?

Fibromyalgia Hazards Found in Church

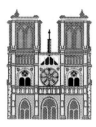

1. Petrified pine pews and kneelers with scant if any padding.

2. Speakers too loud for uninterrupted snoozing.

3. Burning, perfumed incense entering dry nasal and eye membranes.

4. Long, single-file communion lines.

5. Single antique ceiling fan that serves as entire church's climate control system.

6. 30 inch leg room space for 34 inch legs.

7. Noxious mix of smelly cosmetics used liberally by attendees.

8. One toilet for 300 parishioners.

9. 517 page song books that have fallen under the pew.

10. Weekly ritual struggling to remember names of all those familiar faces.

Mispronunciations of Fibromyalgia

1. fi bro my **LAYS** ya

2. fi **BER ALS** ya

3. **FIB** bro my **ALS** ya

4. fi bro my al **GEE** a

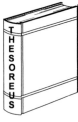

5. fi bro my **ALL GEE**

6. fi **BRALS** ya

7. fi bro my **LALS** ya

8. fi **BER** my **ALS** ya

9. fi bro my a ...WHATEVER

10. fi bro my **AL** ler **GEE**

※   ※   ※

LIMERICKS
and more

※   ※   ※

Said Helen to Doctor McFeat,

"I always feel tired and beat."

He said, "Mrs. Wheelings,

To dodge rundown feelings,

Be careful when crossing the
street."

*   *   *

My symptoms onset with
rapidity

Fibers fast filled with flaccidity

Limbs grow stiff

While sinuses sniff

And brainfog renders stupidity.

I went to my doctor to see

What might be the matter with
me.

"The source of your pain

Lies deep in your brain,"

Mused the medic most
mournfully.

✻   ✻   ✻

My doc first said, "neurotic,"

'Cause my pains were so
sporadic.

But he realized

What I'd surmised

When he spied my muscles
spasmodic.

A woman whose name was Flo

Woke up one day raring to go.

But 'though hours she'd rested

Her muscles protested

And screamed "Oh no, no no NO!"

❋　　❋　　❋

Then there was Jane, poor dearie

Whose way was usually cheery.

But yes, you guessed it,

Her FM has messed it

And now she feels achy and
weary.

A Fibro fellow named Marty

Felt good so decided to party.

He forgot about "pacing"

Sent his pain levels racing

And thus proved he's not such a
smarty!

✴   ✴   ✴

Just spoke with my friend Stu

Who claims "It's only the flu."

But really, Stu dear

It's been more than a year!

Don't you think that's somewhat
of a clue?

Pain, pain, go away

I do not need you today,

Come back another day

Like when I'm dead.

❄   ❄   ❄

Sorry, boss, I cannot give

The presentation today.

My fibromyalgia has affected

My TMJ.

There once was a woman in pain.

But hardly ever did to her
husband complain

For he was her very best supporter

You see he did very much adore
her.

She said to her husband so dear,

"I really don't mean to be drear

But this pain is everywhere except
my ear."

He said, "I'm sorry you're in so
much pain.

To be there for you always is my
aim."

She looked at him with a very big smile

And said, "Honey, I sure do like
your style."

— BHR

There once was a fair lass named Bonnie

Whose twin sister happened to be Connie.

Her twin did say on one gloomy day

"Dear sister why are you so stiff and lame?"

Bonnie did quickly reply, "You see Pain is my name.

Not sleeping is my game.

And besides all that this all over pain and pain in my neck was brought on by a wreck.

What the heck! Now I'm stuck with this Pain-O-myalgia."

— BHR

✳   ✳   ✳

There once was a Bonnie lass

Who sighed "Alas! Alas!

The cause of this pain is the
  rain, is the rain."

So now I must really refrain.

Please go away pain, and play
  in the rain

So this pain I won't have to
  explain.

— BHR

✳   ✳   ✳

✳   ✳   ✳

Pitter patter here comes the rain.

Pitter patter here comes the pain.

April showers bring more than
May flowers.

So hurry away April with all of
your rain and all of your pain.

Just give me May with all of its
flowers with no rain and no pain.

April fool!

— BHR

✳   ✳   ✳

*Thanks to Bonnie H. Robinson, Leicester, NC
for contributions to this chapter.*

WHAT YOU SAY, WHAT YOU MEAN

WHAT YOU SAY: I used to have a photographic memory.

WHAT YOU MEAN: Doctor, my brain is out of film!

WHAT YOU SAY: I used to go on vacations.

WHAT YOU MEAN: The only things that travel now are my pains.

WHAT YOU SAY: I'm not asking for new sympathetic friends.

WHAT YOU MEAN: I really want new sympathetic nerves!

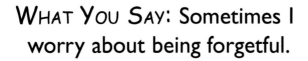

WHAT YOU SAY: Sometimes I worry about being forgetful.

WHAT YOU MEAN: Oh, my gosh, did I remember to unplug the coffee pot before I left?

WHAT YOU SAY: Sir, could you give me directions to downtown?

WHAT YOU MEAN: Sir, could you tell me what planet we are on?

WHAT YOU SAY: I sleep like a baby.

WHAT YOU MEAN: I sleep a while and then wake up and cry a while.

WHAT YOU SAY: I slept like a dream.

WHAT YOU MEAN: My sleep is like nightmare on Elm Street.

FAMOUS LAST WORDS (FLAWS)

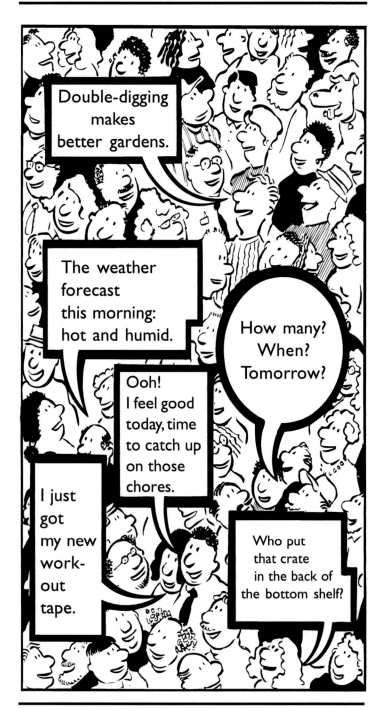

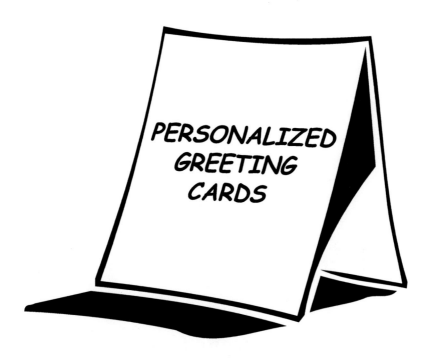

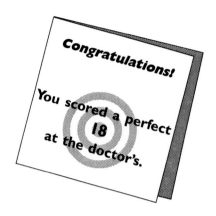

Congratulations!

You scored a perfect 18 at the doctor's.

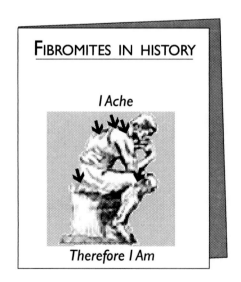

FIBROMITES IN HISTORY

I Ache

Therefore I Am

I know you have an
important event happening

I forgot which one though.

Please check which one
applies...
☐ **Happy Birthday!**
☐ *Happy Anniversary*
☐ Congratulations!
☐ Other

Flare-up
Condolences
Remember: a flare-up
is like a good meal...

In time
this too shall pass.

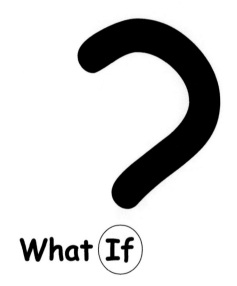

What If

What if the maker of stairs had fibro?

Instead of stairs like:

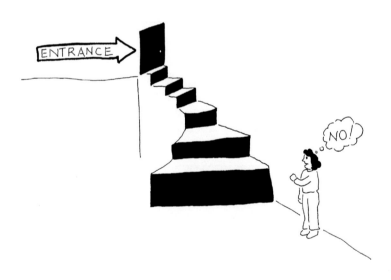

They would have looked like:

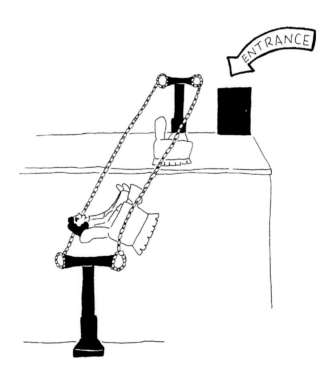

What if the creator of the cartoon
thought bubble had FMS?
Instead of cartoon bubbles looking like:

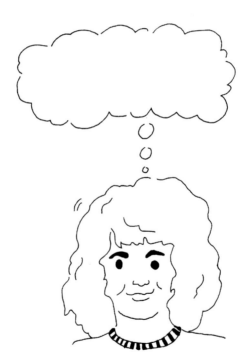

They would have looked like:

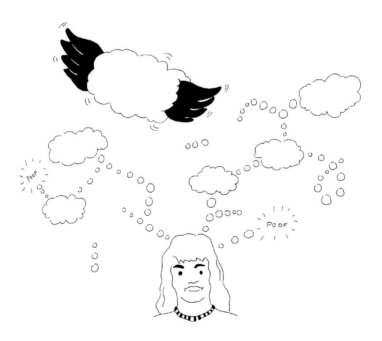

If Richard Simmons had FMS with IBS, instead of his diet plan looking like:

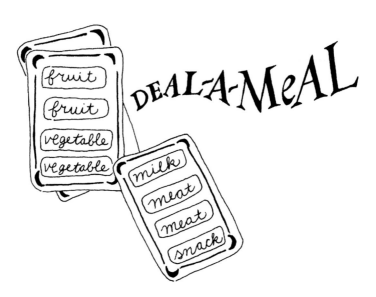

It would have been:

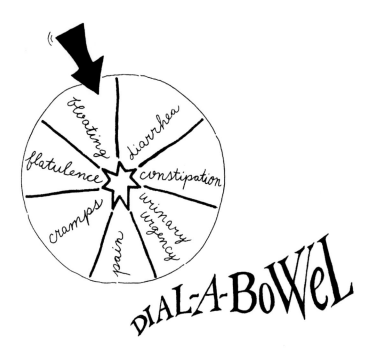

What if the inventor of the sleeping bag had fibromyalgia and brain fog? Instead of the sleeping bag looking like:

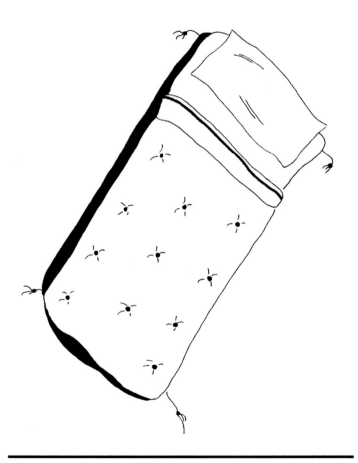

It would have looked like this:

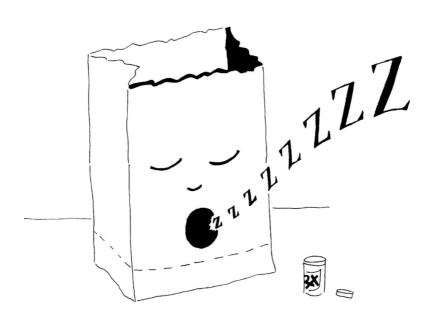

PAINECDOTES

Fibromyalgia causes us to experience many things — especially pain. This section includes a variety of experiences and reflections relating to life with fibromyalgia. The names are fictional, and any reference to any individual is purely coincidental.

Bonnie McBride read about tennis ball acupressure in a fibromyalgia book. Deciding a tennis ball was too small for *her* fibromyalgia pains, she chose a much larger, hard foam ball. A shrewd consumer, she refused to fork out the 99-cent price until certain the technique worked. Bonnie hiked up to the counter, positioned the ball between her hip and the counter, and squirmed around until the ball "hit" a trigger point. Well, that felt so good she decided to work on another spot in her hip. And another. Finally she looked up and spotted a man at the end of the aisle. He was looking straight at Bonnie and grinning from ear to ear. Grabbing an armload of "priceless therapeutic devices" she dashed for the cashier counter. After all, some things about fibromyalgia cannot be explained to just any lay person.

While enlightening a graduate class about an event in the Industrial Education Building, known as the I-E-D Building, I mistakenly said "I-U-D Building." I didn't notice, though. That is, until one of the few females in the class screeched "Barbara, you said 'I-U-D.'" There's always someone around willing to help you get full credit for every blunder! This moment of shame happened after my fibromyalgia diagnosis but before I'd learned about the noun-retrieval problems many of us have. *sigh*

A lady from another state told me she understood perfectly. She led incoming freshmen and parents on library tours during summer orientations. To one group she proudly announced the library is a federal suppository library instead of a federal depository library. Afterward, one father told her some folks considered their entire state a suppository.

I often wear my fibromyalgia survivor T-shirt to support group meetings. The shirt sports huge red spots marking characteristic tender point locations. One lady came up behind me and, with more force than I could have mustered, poked the two spots on my rear end and said, "I have these two." The spots are indeed in the correct place. When I landed, I thought, "She must not have them or surely she would know better than to inflict such pain on another!"

I attended a conference for fibromyalgia patients in San Antonio in 1995. The day before the conference I arrived in town in plenty of time to walk around and get my bearings. Yeah, right! Well, I tried. My two roommates arrived quite late — Susan hailing from south Florida and Karen from Tennessee. We were all hungry so my recently acquired knowledge from my reconnaissance stroll came in handy. We traipsed directly to the food court in the mall only to find BARS firmly in place. The food court was locked up tight. We were awfully hungry. Music resounding around the River Walk area and people milling to and fro caused us to believe surely a source of nourishment could be found. We continued our search.

At last we found a restaurant. We seated ourselves with great expectation of culinary delights. After a while we noticed we were the only table of females in the place. We noticed that the waitresses were scantily clad. But we were awfully hungry.

Waitresses flitted about — but not to our table. The manager, the only male who appeared to be working in the place, approached our table, looked at each of us, then said, "Are you ladies here for the dog show?" Susan was sporting a poodle-esque 'do with her hair in a bun at the top of her head. We tried our best to keep our composure. But of all the insults! The nerve! We ordered, were served, and staggered back to our rooms.

The next day we discovered there actually was a huge pedigreed dog show in town.

My last night in town my roommates, Susan and Karen were leaving. Occasionally over the days of the conference, Mary announced she was heading to her room to work on the manuscript of her fibromyalgia book. Economizing, I asked Debbie if I could share her room that last night after our roomies departed. She agreed under one condition: the hotel change the mattress on which Mary had slept. Each time Mary so much as wiggled, her mattress "crunched," disturbing Debbie's repose.

Maxine ordered the mattress-ectomy and I moved in. We later decided the crunching came from drafts of Mary's book stashed for safekeeping!

❖

We installed a used hot tub on our carport. Soaking in moist heat greatly helps our pain. Three buttons labeled "jets," "blower," and "light" make operation easy. Liz attends our support group meetings. Her pain level seemed so high I invited her to come over and try out the hot tub. First time she came over, we both got in and soaked until we became two happy hunks of protoplasm. The next time she came over, I was busy and she soaked alone. The third time, I was finishing up something and joined her after she'd started soaking.

Noticing only the jets were on, I activated the blowers and commented I liked the full massaging effect from both jets and blowers. Liz remarked she did too.

When I wondered aloud why she pre-
ferred both and only used one of them,
she sheepishly admitted she'd noticed
there was much less motion but thought
maybe something was broken.

I watched the USA lady gymnasts vault
into history. What talent! What courage!
But surely antics necessary to get off the
doctor's examining table with a minimum
of pain merits gold rating, too. Imagine:
points for form, degree of difficulty, origi-
nality, and a stuck landing.

♪ PARODIES: FIBROMYALGIA SONGS

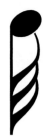

Fibro Crud
Tune: Jingle Bells

A few years back, it seems,
I thought I felt a twinge,
My doc I went to see,
He said, "No need to cringe!"

"We all get aches and pains.
No need to get upset,"
He said, "No need to come again!"
Now, that doctor was all wet!

OH!

Fibro crud, fibro crud,
Muscles now all ache.
I thought the pain would go away
but it is here to stay.
Fibro crud, fibro crud,
Muscles now all ache.
I thought the pain would go away
but it is here to stay.

Twelve Years of Fibro
Tune: The Twelve Days of Christmas

In the first year of fibro,
my doctor said to me
There's noth-thi-ing wro-ong, you see.

In the second year of fibro,
my doctor said to me
Te-ests are normal.
So there's noth-thi-ing wro-ong, you see.

In the third year of fibro,
my doctor said to me
You feel tired.
Te-ests are normal.
So there's noth-thi-ing wro-ong, you see.

In the fourth year of fibro,
my doctor said to me
Pain in your back.
You feel tired.

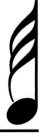

Te-ests are normal.
So there's noth-thi-ing wro-ong,
you see.

In the fifth year of fibro,
my doctor said to me
YOU SLEEP NO MORE.
Pain in your back.
You feel tired.
Te-ests are normal.
So there's noth-thi-ing wro-ong, you see.

In the sixth year of fibro,
my doctor said to me
Bowels irritated.
YOU SLEEP NO MORE.
Pain in your back.
You feel tired.
Te-ests are normal.
So there's noth-thi-ing wro-ong, you see.

In the seventh year of fibro,
my doctor said to me
Neck is sore.
Bowels irritated.
YOU SLEEP NO MORE.

Pain in your back.
You feel tired.
Te-ests are normal.
So there's noth-thi-ing wro-ong, you see.

In the eighth year of fibro,
my doctor said to me
Head is a'hurting.
Neck is sore.
Bowels irritated.
YOU SLEEP NO MORE.
Pain in your back.
You feel tired.
Te-ests are normal.
So there's noth-thi-ing wro-ong, you see.

In the ninth year of fibro,
my doctor said to me
Hips are a'aching.
Head is a'hurting.
Neck is sore.
Bowels irritated.
YOU SLEEP NO MORE.
Pain in your back.

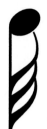
You feel tired.
Te-ests are normal.
So there's noth-thi-ing wro-ong,
you see.

In the tenth year of fibro,
my doctor said to me
Muscles are a'twitching.
Hips are a'aching.
Head is a'hurting.
Neck is sore.
Bowels irritated.
YOU SLEEP NO MORE.
Pain in your back.
You feel tired.
Te-ests are normal.
So there's noth-thi-ing wro-ong, you see.

In the eleventh year of fibro,
my doctor said to me.
Brain is a'blurring.
Muscles are a'twitching.
Hips are a'aching.
Head is a'hurting.
Neck is sore.
Bowels irritated.

YOU SLEEP NO MORE.
Pain in your back.
You feel tired.
Te-ests are normal.
So there's noth-thi-ing wro-ong, you see.

In the twelfth year of fibro,
my doctor said to me
Body is a'failing.
Brain is a'blurring.
Muscles are a'twitching.
Hips are a'aching.
Head is a'hurtin.g
Neck is sore.
Bowels irritated.
YOU SLEEP NO MORE.
Pain in your back.
You feel tired.
Te-ests are normal.
So there's noth-thi-ing wro-ong, you see.

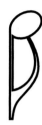

Myofascial Pain
Tune: Kum Bah Yah

Myofaschial pain, please release;
Myofaschial pain, please release;
Myofaschial pain, please release;
Oh, P.T., please release.

Gastrocnemius aches,
release these please;
Piriformis aches,
release these please;
My trapezius aches,
release these please;
Oh, P.T., release these please.

Muscles now at ease,
they've been released;
Muscles now at ease,
they've been released;
Muscles now at ease,
they've been released;
Oh, P.T., they've been released.

The Flu That Never Ends
Tune: The Song That Never Ends

This is the flu that never ends
It goes on and on, my friend.
One day it start-ed hurting, not
knowing what it was
And it will go on hurting, forever,
just because.... (REPEAT)

Jessica Hitch, Garland, Texas assisted
with these lyrics.

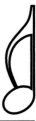

I Wish I Were A CNP[1]
Tune: I Wish I Were . . .

I wish I were a Cee En Pee-ee
That is what I'd really like to be-ee-eee
'Cause if I were a Cee En Pee-ee
Nothing woo-ould be-ee wrong
with me.

[1] CNP = chronically normal person

My Fibro Had A First Pain
Tune: My Bologna Has A First Name

My body had a first pain
It was in my right shoulder.
My body had some more pains
That made me feel older.
I lack the stuff that makes cells grow
Each day I ache from head to toe
'Cause doc sez I've got a combo
of M. P. S. and fi-eye-bro.

The Ants Go Marchin'
'Neath My Skin
(A Tribute to the "Phantom Itch")
Tune: The Ants Go Marchin'

The ants go marching 'neath my
skin. Yee-oow, yee-oow.
The ants go marching 'neath my
skin. Yee-oow, yee-oow.
The ants go marching 'neath my skin.
I scratch, they move, I itch again.
And the ants go marching,
Up, to my head, and back down,
to my feet.

The ants go marching up my leg.
Yee-oow, yee-oow.
The ants go marching up my leg.
Yee-oow, yee-oow.
The ants go marching up my leg.
They itch so much, I start to beg.
And the ants go marching,
Up, to my head, and back down,
to my feet.

The ants go marching down my
arm. Yee-oow, yee-oow.
The ants go marching down my
arm. Yee-oow, yee-oow.
The ants go marching down
my arm.
I am alarmed I've done some harm.
And the ants go marching,
Up, to my head, and back down,
to my feet.

The ants go marching o'er my nose.
Yee-oow, yee-oow.
The ants go marching o'er my nose.
Yee-oow, yee-oow.
The ants go marching o'er my nose.
I know not why it's me they chose.
And the ants go marching,
Up, to my head, and back down,
to my feet.

The ants go marching 'cross my
back. Yee-oow, yee-oow.
The ants go marching 'cross my
back. Yee-oow, yee-oow.
The ants go marching 'cross my back.

I've scratched so much
I've now lost track.
And the ants go marching,
Up, to my head, and back down,
to my feet.

The ants go marching 'neath my
skin. Yee-oow, yee-oow.
The ants go marching 'neath my
skin. Yee-oow, yee-oow.
The ants go marching 'neath my skin.
I scratch, they move, I itch again.
And the ants go marching,
Up, to my head, and back down, to
my feet.
<Softer> Up, to my head, and back
down, to my feet.
<Barely audible> Up, to my head, and
back down, to my feet.

Ruby Morrison and Rachel Morrison of
Brookwood, Alabama and
Norma Shaw, Gore Springs, Mississippi
assisted with these lyrics.

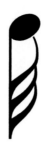

Fibro Song
Tune: This Old Man

I love you, you love me
We've got Fibro-crud you see
 With the brain-fog, dizziness, aches
 and pa-ain too
  Fibro-crud will make you blue.

Now I take, lots of pills
 But I've got some symptoms still
  I've got brain-fog, dizziness, aches
 and pa-ain too
  Fibro-crud will make you blue.

Now I've lost, my car key
 I don't know where it might be
  I've got brain-fog, dizziness, aches
 and pa-ain too
  Fibro-crud will make you blue.

When I walk, like I'm drunk
Things I hit sometimes go thunk
  I've got brain-fog, dizziness, aches
  and pa-ain too
    Fibro-crud will make you blue.

The real test, is M P S.
 Muscles tighten but never rest.
  I've got brain-fog, dizziness, aches
  and pa-ain too
    Fibro-crud will make you blue.

All my cells, are clogged within
 Now I take Guai-fen-e-sin.
  I've got brain-fog, dizziness, aches
  and pa-ain too
    Fibro-crud will make you blue.

It's so sad, brain-fog's bad
 Can't remember the words I had
  I've got duh, duh, duh-duh-duh, duh
  duh du-uh doo
    Fibro-crud will make you blue.

MiscellPAINey

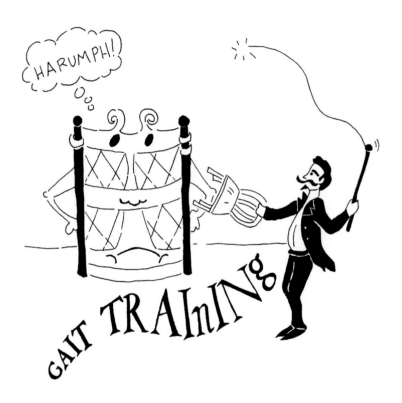

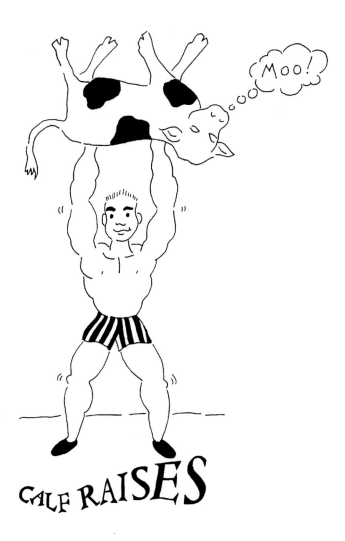

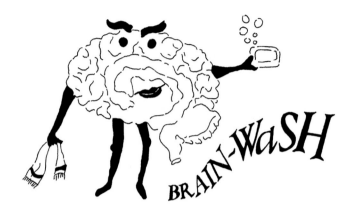

BRAIN-WaSH

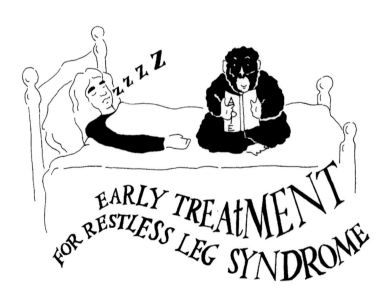

EARLY TREAtMENT FOR RESTLESS LEG SYNDROME

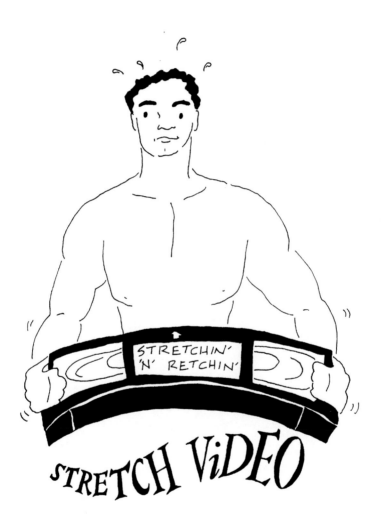

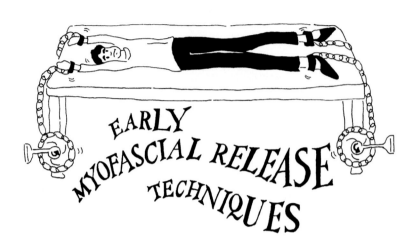

EARLY MYOFASCIAL RELEASE TECHNIQUES

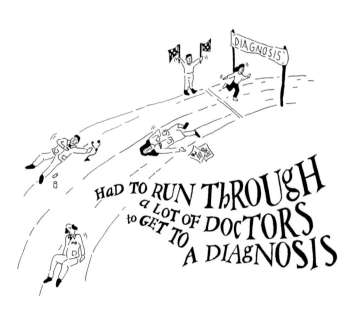

HaD TO RUN ThROUGH a LOT OF DOCTORS to GET TO A DIAGNOSIS

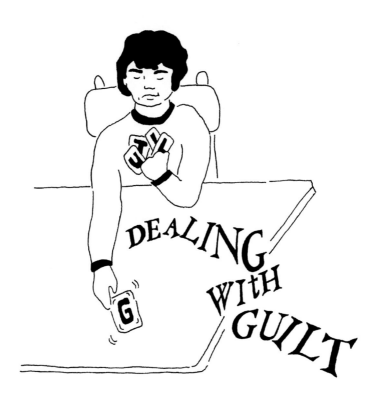

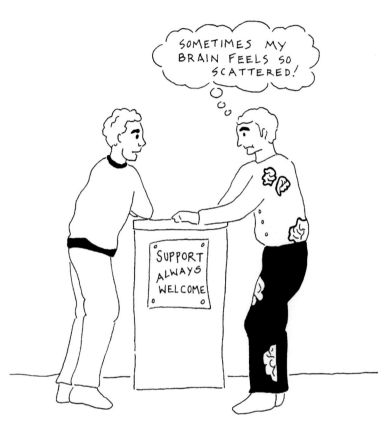

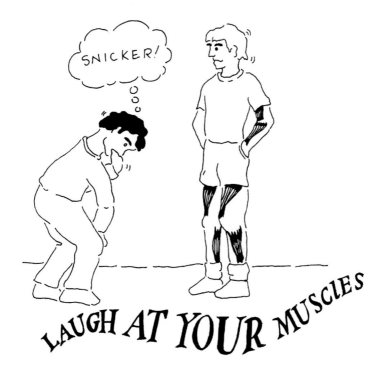

How Bad Is My Pain?

MY PAIN IS SO BAD THAT...
    A hot poker tickles me.

MY PAIN IS SO BAD THAT...
    Semi trucks swerve to avoid
    running over me.

MY PAIN IS SO BAD THAT...
    Others take narcotics when
    they see me.

MY PAIN IS SO BAD THAT...
    The sound of a dental drill is
    actually soothing to me.

MY PAIN IS SO BAD THAT...
    In the *Complete Encyclopedia
    of Pain*, I am Volumes 7–12.

MY PAIN IS SO BAD THAT...
    Hungry mosquitoes avoid me.

MY PAIN IS SO BAD THAT...
>When I visit someone in the hospital I receive Get Well cards.

MY PAIN IS SO BAD THAT...
>I set off ambulance sirens when I walk past them.

MY PAIN IS SO BAD THAT...
>My last nerve block numbed my doctor.

MY PAIN IS SO BAD THAT...
>My dog brings me medications.

MY PAIN IS SO BAD THAT...
>My shingles are staying at a motel.

MY PAIN IS SO BAD THAT...
>I have been declared the "World's Only Living Martyr."

MY PAIN IS SO BAD THAT...
>Kidney stones fear me.

More Books for
"Helping You Live Life to the Fullest"

If you enjoyed *Laugh at Your Muscles II,* you will be interested in other resources from Anadem Publishing. We are devoted to providing health information to assist individuals with chronic conditions in taking charge of their recovery and in getting the most out of life.

Fibromyalgia: Managing the Pain
by Mark J. Pellegrino, M.D.
Dr. Pellegrino delivers a comprehensive guide to the syndrome. It is the ideal book for the recently diagnosed FMS patient from the doctor who treats fibromyalgia patients and has it himself.

The Fibromyalgia Survivor
by Mark J. Pellegrino, M.D.
The Fibromyalgia Survivor is packed with good advice and tips on every aspect of living your life to the fullest. You get the specific step-by-step "how to's" for daily living. Plus, you learn *Fibronomics,* the four key principles that help you minimize your pain in every situation.

Understanding Post-Traumatic Fibromyalgia
by Mark J. Pellegrino, M.D.
Everyone with post-traumatic fibromyalgia will benefit from reading the first book focusing exclusively on this condition. Dr. Pellegrino presents the medical perspective on post-traumatic fibromyalgia and how it differs from other forms of fibromyalgia.

The Fibromyalgia Supporter
by Mark J. Pellegrino, M.D.
Dr. Pellegrino explains how it feels to have fibromyalgia, how you can get the support you deserve, and how you and your loved one can enjoy life together. Dr. Pellegrino combines compassion, humor and empathy with his professional expertise to provide specific steps to achieve a real "partnership" in dealing with fibromyalgia.

Laugh at Your Muscles
by Mark J. Pellegrino, M.D.
An easy, light read that you can enjoy and benefit from.

Chronic Fatigue Syndrome: Charting Your Course to Recovery
by Mary E. O'Brien, M.D.
Mary O'Brien, M.D., shares her personal experience in overcoming many of the debilitating effects of chronic fatigue syndrome. In an easy-to-read, nonmechanical format, Dr. O'Brien shares advice on treatment options and self-help steps that will help you rebuild your stamina.

TMJ — Its Many Faces
by Wesley Shankland, D.D.S., M.S.
Fibromyalgia patients frequently suffer from TMJ disorders and orofacial pain. Dr. Shankland's book is filled with step-by-step instructions on how to relieve TMJ, head, neck and facial pain.

Pills Aren't Enough
by Cody Wasner, M.D.
    Pills Aren't Enough by Cody Wasner, M.D. , is a special kind of book — fictional stories of unforgettable characters help you identify your own emotions. Written by a doctor who himself has come to terms with a chronic condition, *Pills Aren't Enough* inspires thought and reflection. To enrich the process of emotional healing, Dr. Wasner provides you a second section with thought-provoking exercises to enhance your self-discovery.

 Anadem Publishing **Helping You Live Life to the Fullest**

Order Your Books Today!
— 30 Day Money Back Guarantee —

For fastest service, call 1•(800)•633-0055

Qty	Title	Price (US$)	Ohio Price*	Total
	Fibromyalgia: Managing The Pain	$12.45	$13.17	
	The Fibromyalgia Survivor	19.50	20.62	
	Understanding Post-Traumatic Fibromyalgia	16.25	17.18	
	The Fibromyalgia Supporter	15.50	16.39	
	Laugh At Your Muscles	5.95	6.29	
	Laugh At Your Muscles II	5.95	6.29	
	CFS: Charting Your Course to Recovery	14.25	15.07	
	TMJ — Its Many Faces	19.50	20.62	
	Pills Aren't Enough	$18.50	$19.62	

Shipping and Handling

For 1 book, add $3.50
2–4 books, add $7.00
5–6 books, add $10
7+, please call
Priority Mail, add $2.50

*Ohio price includes 5.75% state sales tax

Subtotal ___

Add shipping and handling (see chart at left) ___

❑ Enclosed is my check, made payable to Anadem, Inc.

❑ Charge my credit card: ❑ **VISA**   ❑ **MasterCard**

TOTAL ___

Card No. _____ Exp. _____

Signature _____

Name _____

Address _____

City _____ State ____ Zip _____ Phone ( ) _____

Anadem Publishing 3620 North High Street • Columbus, OH • 43214
1-800-633-0055 • FAX (614) 262-6630 • http://www.anadem.com

You can count on Anadem Publishing to keep you informed of the newest, most advanced ideas to help you get the most out of life. Let us know if you want to be placed on our mailing list to be notified of new resources. And come visit us at our website!

http://www.anadem.com

Laugh at Your Muscles II

Laugh at Your Muscles II

Barbara Dawkins
Mark J. Pellegrino, M.D.

Anadem Publishing, Inc.
Columbus, Ohio 43214
614•262•2539
800•633•0055
http://www.anadem.com

Printed in the U.S.A.
ISBN 1-890018-15-5

The material in *Laugh at Your Muscles II* is presented for informational purposes only. It is not meant to be a substitute for proper medical care by your doctor. You need to consult with your doctor for diagnosis and treatment.